Starting today, you define your future.

The information in this guide should not be used for diagnosing or treating a health problem. Not all diet and exercise plans suit everyone. Consult your licensed healthcare provider before starting a diet, taking any form of prescription medication, or embarking on any fitness or weight training program.

The creator and content provider disclaim any liability or loss in connection with the information and advice provided here.

By reading this guide, you agree to the terms listed above.

You have taken the first step to becoming the person you dream of becoming. You want to lose weight. Thoughts of it consume your mind every second, every minute, every hour, every day, every year. Today, that is going to change. I am going to teach you how to modify your thoughts and your eating, and lead you to getting the body of your dreams. Starting today, right now, understand that you are in control. Your days will no longer be filled with sadness and despair and feelings of misery. Your days are going to be filled with elation, anticipation, and delight. You are starting on a venture that is going to take you wherever you want to go.

The steps in my plan are not traditional. Many of them may seem unimportant. The key to making my plan work is to follow every step regardless of how insignificant it may seem to you. Everybody is different on how soon they will see weight loss. It can be as soon as three days or as long as ten days. Do not get discouraged. If you follow each step, you will lose weight. Even if you do not see it on the scale as soon as you'd like, know that change is happening in you and one day you are going to step on the scale and realize you have lost weight. You are going to come to the realization that you can control your weight, and that my plan does work. You are going to realize that you truly are capable of attaining the body of your dreams.

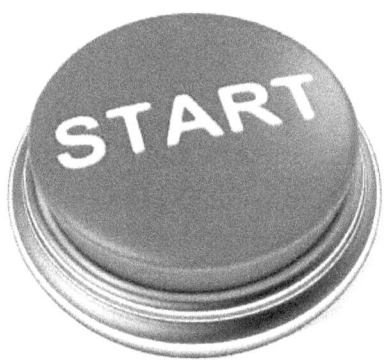

Step 1: Visualize the end result.

Get a picture of someone whose body you admire. Someone who has the ideal body you dream of having. Keep the picture nearby you at all times. Feel like a creeper? Don't. It is your motivation. It is a reminder to you of what it is that you are on your way to becoming.

Look at the picture frequently. See yourself transforming into who you want to be. Know it is going to happen. You are going to make it happen. It is your goal, your dream. You are going to attain it and make it come true. Today, you are taking control of how your body looks. Your body is the clay. You are the sculptor. You are going to design your body to make it look exactly how you want it to be.

Determine today that not only are you going to have the body like that person in the picture, yours is going to be even better. See yourself walking down the red carpet at an important event. By the time you get to the end of that carpet, you are going to be the person you want to be. Your goals and dreams are important to you and you are going to get noticed for reaching them.

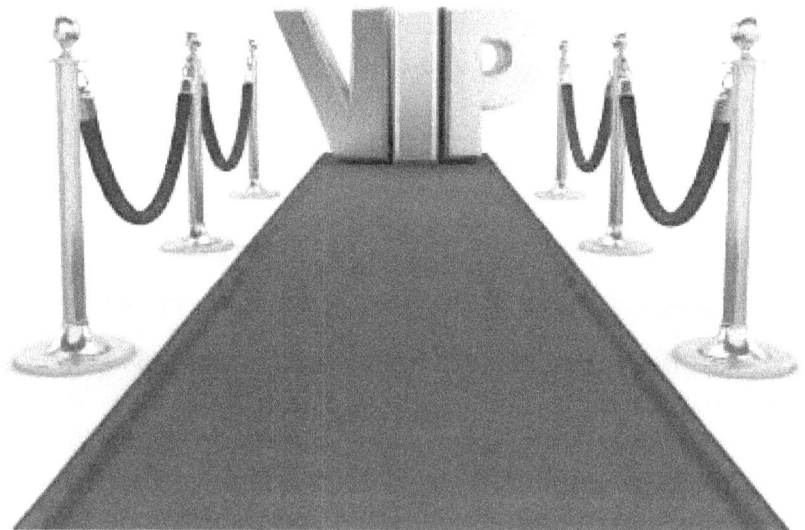

6

Step 2: Lose Weight Instantly

I'm talking about mental weight. Whatever it is that is always in the back of your mind weighing you down. Maybe a business deal went bad. You lost all of your money in the stock market. Somebody broke your heart. Your parents make you feel like you never measure up to their expectations. Whatever it is, let it go. Wallowing in self pity makes you non-productive, anti-social, and induces comfort eating. We all know one person or event that has had a huge negative impact on our life. To you, it is like quicksand. Every time you see that person or think about what happened, your mind starts racing, emitting thought after thought after thought after thought.

These thoughts surround you, consume you, and engulf you until you're spinning out of control and drowning in feelings of helplessness, sorrow, and failure. Dwelling over and over about "what if" is a waste of your time, exhausting, and weighs you down. It prevents you from being the best you can be. The fact that you are reading this right now indicates that you are not happy with the way you feel and look. You are ready for change. You are ready to move beyond where you are now. You cannot control what people do to you or what life throws at you. What you can control is what you do to your body. You have total control of how you look. Stop being a victim. Replace those feelings of helplessness with power. You have the power to change yourself. Replace your sorrow with joy. You

7

have a lot to be happy about. You are taking control of your life back. You are on your way to victory. Today, you're doing something to change it all…your mind, your body, your life.

Don't go near the "quicksand". Don't allow yourself to even think about it for a second. Fill your mind with thoughts about how excited you are that you are on your way to a new you. You aren't going to allow things to get you down anymore. You are in control. You are on your way up, on your way to the top. Yesterday is gone.

Tomorrow is arriving. So are you. The new you will be arriving soon. Everyday that passes, you are closer to becoming the person you long to be. Everyday is a step up to help you closer to reaching your dream.

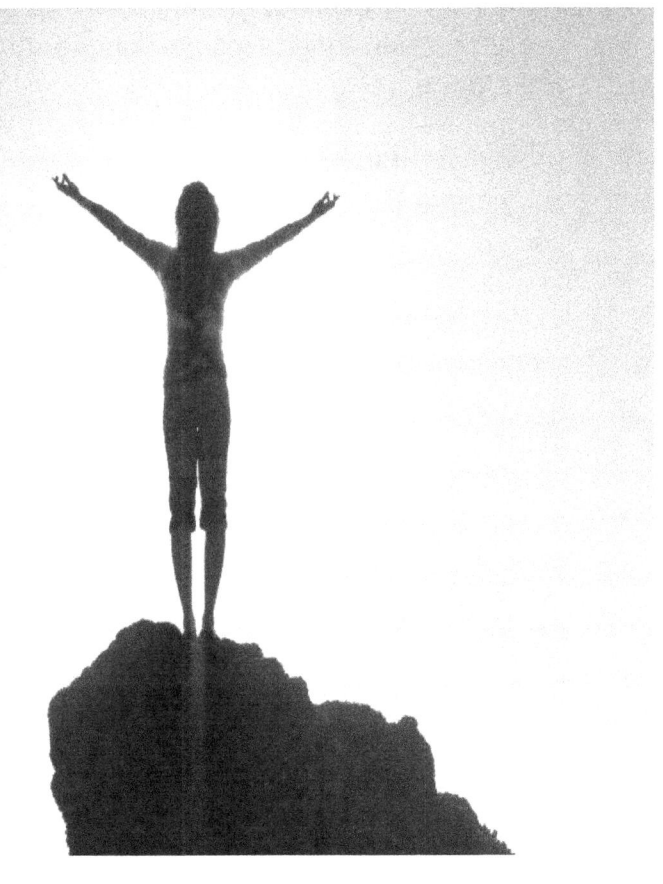

Step 3: Think of your life in calendar format.

Get a calendar. Chances are that up to now, you have just passively existed, making a few feeble attempts every now and then to lose weight. Everyday you wake up, eat destructively, hate yourself for eating destructively, feel like garbage, then go to sleep knowing that tomorrow will be exactly the same. Put an "X" on today's date. Starting today, you are taking back control of your life. Look at the date 10 days from today. Draw a ⅄ there. In ten days, you will start seeing the results of your efforts. In twenty days, your friends will start noticing that you're losing weight. In thirty days, you will look back at the date with the "X" in the box and rejoice at how far you've come. This may seem like an insignificant step. On the contrary, it is extremely significant. Looking at a calendar helps to keep the passage of time in a perspective that is tangible. You are not a helpless victim just enduring the passage of time. You are in control of what you do each and every day. Everyday that goes by you are a step closer to reaching your goal.

10

Step 4: Think like a soldier.

Starting today, you are on a secret mission. I know that you're excited about your new venture, but keep it to yourself. Don't exclaim at the dinner table that you're officially on a new diet. Don't brag to your friends that you've found the ultimate diet plan that is going to change your life. As much as I'd love for them to buy my 10-step plan, this is between you and yourself. You are doing this for you.

Only you know how you feel and what you need to do to be happy. Telling them will likely put them on defense. I am not sure why, but it is human nature. Out of sheer insecurity and jealousy, some will try to sabotage your efforts, discourage you, or simply tell you to stop being so vain about how you look. Just know that you have started on a journey that is going to lead you to a happier life. You are going to look better and feel better. Soon, your friends will start seeing your results and be showering you with compliments. Your transition may even motivate them to change their lives, too. Your family and friends have the biggest impact on what you do everyday. Their lives are not changing. They are still going to bake cookies in the house, serve ice cream for dessert, and munch on nachos during the movie. There are going to be temptations and obstacles. Think of yourself as a soldier on a mission. There is

11

one objective. That objective is to destroy the enemy. That enemy is your fat. Stay on course. You are in control. All of those temptations are like bullets trying to detain you from reaching your goal. Stay strong.

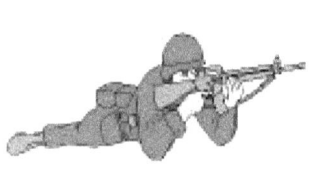 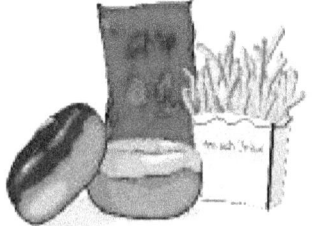

Step 5: Discover your new favorite number.

Today, you are going to unveil a number that is going to change your life. With my plan, you do not have to give up anything that you love to eat. You just have to eat it in moderation. Use this formula to calculate the number of calories you can consume each day and still lose weight.

Women: 11 x your dream weight = your new favorite number

Men: 12 x your dream weight = your new favorite number

Don't be intimidated. Don't decide that you have just wasted your money on this plan. You can do this. You want to do it. You want to make change happen. You are making change happen by reading this.
Remember this number. Make it your new favorite number. It is going to change your life.

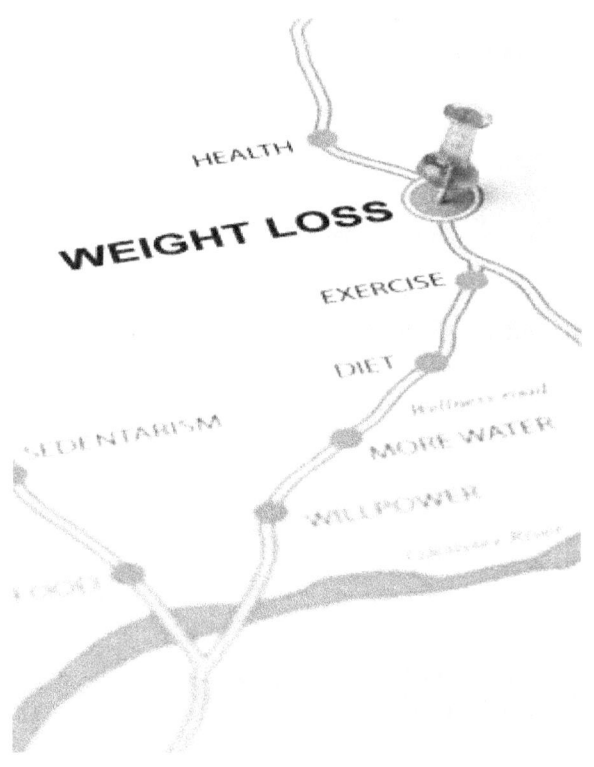

Step 6: Keep track of what you consume.

The closer you stay to your new favorite number, the faster you will see results. The healthier the foods you eat, the faster you will see results. I am not going to tell you to only eat meat that has been prepared on the grill. I am not going to list healthy foods that you're "allowed" to eat. If you're like me, you've seen these lists and ran to the grocery store to buy them. You resolve that you are only going to eat the list of "approved" foods for the rest of your life. You excitedly arrange them carefully in the cupboards and fridge so you can easily access them. Your friends invite you to go out to dinner the first day, so you do, but with the adamant intention that you'll start your new diet tomorrow. The second day, you "pig out" one last time just to get rid of any junk food that is still in the house so that you won't be tempted to eat it tomorrow when you start your diet. The third day, it seems like way too much work to go outside to grill the chicken, so you order pizza instead. The fourth day, you have a busy day at work. You're running late so you stop and pick up fast food on the way home. By the fifth day, the only one eating the "approved" fruit is the annoying little fruit fly. The "approved" vegetables are wilted and the only reason you take the "approved" chicken out of the fridge is because you can't take the smell of it disintegrating.

Changing your eating habits is not easy to do. With my plan, you do not have to give up anything that you

15

love to eat. Obviously, you should try to cut back on the amount of junk food you consume.

Grilled chicken or fish are good choices. Fruits are good for you, but many are high in calories. Eat them in moderation. If you love bread, try to switch from white to wheat. When you use sugar, instead of white pure cane sugar, use turbinado sugar or "sugar in the raw". Try snacking on uncooked vegetables or air popped popcorn. You don't have to eat healthy all the time on this plan. However, you should try to be more conscientious of the choices that you make. Choices are opportunity. Opportunity enables you to benefit. From now on, resolve that you are going to benefit from the choices you make. You control what you put into your body.

If you're reading this guide, I am going to assume that you're overweight. If you're overweight, you are probably consuming way more calories per day than you should be.   It didn't matter to you before, but now that you've begun your transformation, you do care. You are looking forward to seeing the results of your efforts.

It is easy to track your calories. Once you get into the habit of being aware of what you're consuming, it becomes second nature. Most food from the grocery store has the caloric value on its label. There are many books available that you can keep on hand for reference. You can do a GOOGLE® search to check how many calories each food has. If you have a smartphone, there are many apps that will help you keep track of your caloric intake.

16

Initially, keep track of absolutely everything you eat and drink and track how many calories you consume each day. Try to stay as close as possible to your new favorite number. You are in control of your progress. You control how quickly you get to your goal.

As you progress, you will want to start eating healthier. You start to care about what you put into your body. The snowball effect kicks in. First, you decide to switch from white bread to wheat bread for your salami sandwich. Then, one day, you get rid of the salami and have tuna. You start seeing results. You get so excited you may start skipping the bread and just eat the tuna. But you're happy about it. You don't feel deprived. You feel empowered. You realize that you are in control. You have the power to make change happen.

You choose to eat healthy because it is taking you where you want to go. You are in control, and it feels good.

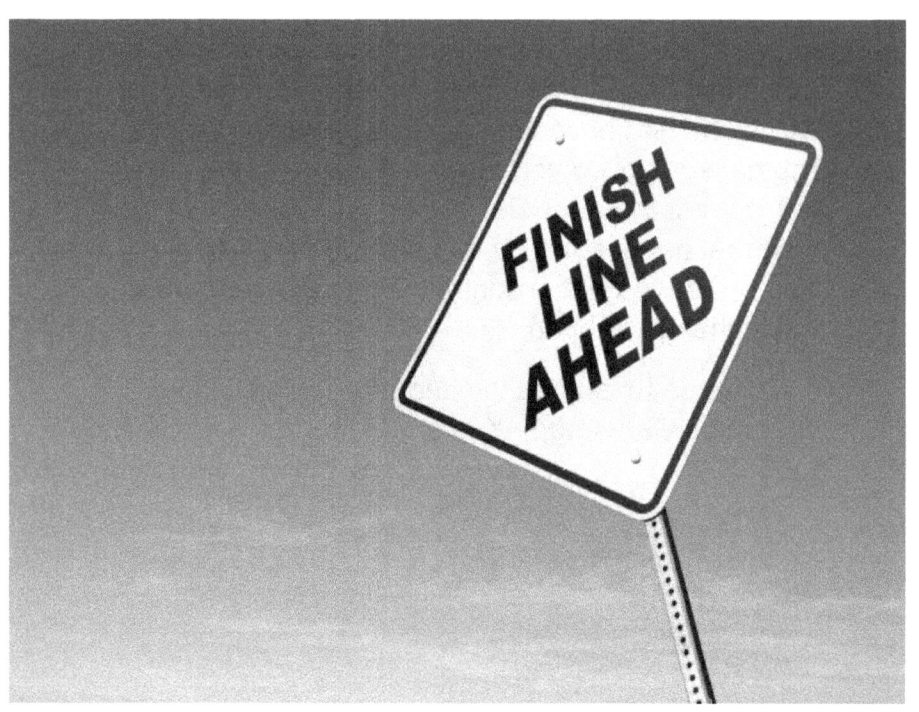

Step 7: Eat Blueberries and Yogurt.

You must consume at least one handful of blueberries between 10:30 a.m. and noon everyday. I don't know why this works, but it does. I have skipped this step and the weight loss stops. I have eaten them earlier or later than those hours and the weight loss stops. You can have a blueberry muffin if you'd rather, just be sure to count the calories. A medium size blueberry muffin has about 350 calories. This step may seem ridiculous to you. I wish I could elaborate on it more, but there is nothing else to say. Trust me, it works.

The last thing you eat each day must be a 6 ounce serving of yogurt. It can be any kind of yogurt that you like, just be sure that it has the active culture L. acidophilus. You do not have to add the calories of the yogurt in your daily total. Again, when I skipped this step, the weight loss stopped.

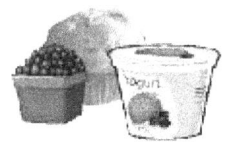

19

Step 8: Don't eat after 6:00 pm.

The most important reason for this is that it helps to establish that you are truly in control of your eating. Most snacking is done while you're sitting on the couch watching television or out with your friends. Today, you are going to make a conscious decision that you are not going to eat after 6:00 p.m. Make this a solemn rule in your life. You may not realize it, but when you sit and munch on snacks while watching television or while you're socializing, it is not because you are hungry. It is just something to do. You see a bowl of chips, you eat them. Your friend buys appetizers for the whole table to share, you eat them. A candy bar is on the kitchen counter, you eat it. Relax, stuff your face, have a few drinks. No harm done, right?

WRONG. The average person does this on a nightly basis. It is destructive behavior. You are done being destructive. You have switched occupations. You are into construction now. You are building yourself up. You are creating a brand new you. When you settle on the couch for the evening ready to watch a movie, don't bring a snack to munch on. You are done with that kind of behavior. That is something the old you would do. You don't want to be that person anymore. You don't want to trudge to bed feeling defeated, stuffed, and suffering from a sugar coma. You are going to choose to go to bed feeling triumphant about your eating for the day. You want to go to bed knowing that another day has passed and you are closer to reaching your dream, the dream of your life.

20

This may take a while getting used to. If you must snack after 6:00 p.m., have air popped popcorn with no butter or raw vegetables. Once you get used to it, you will not be hungry during the evening.

You don't feel like you're starving. You will start to feel really good because you're not stuffing yourself with "fat building" garbage food. For the first time in a long time, you're getting rid of fat. You're getting skinny.

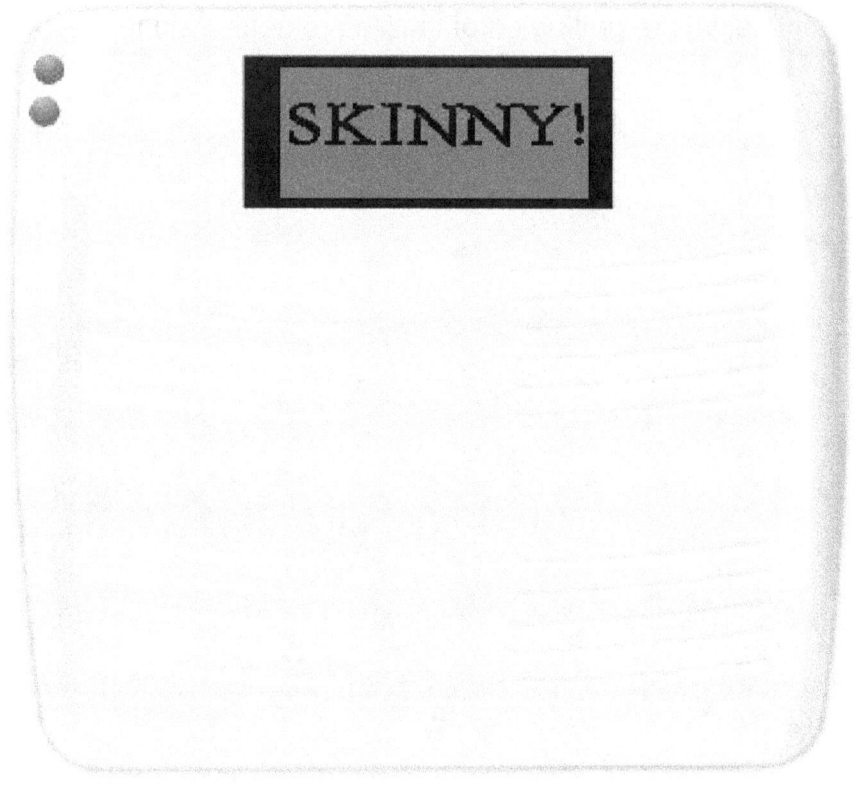

Step 9: Sit in a sauna for at least twenty minutes everyday.

Don't think that you can just ignore this step and decide that it doesn't apply to you because you do not have a sauna. This is essential to losing weight. Sitting in a sauna for twenty minutes can burn up to 300 calories. In addition, it flushes toxins out of the body, is good for your skin, and gets rid of water weight. Believe it or not, you will start to look forward to the time you spend in the sauna. It is peaceful and relaxing. It is a great escape from a busy, hectic and stressful day. Find a health club nearby that has a sauna and buy a membership. Don't despair, it is money well spent. Once you've gotten your eating under control, you will want to start exercising to "tweak" and "fine tune" your body exactly to how you want it to be.

23

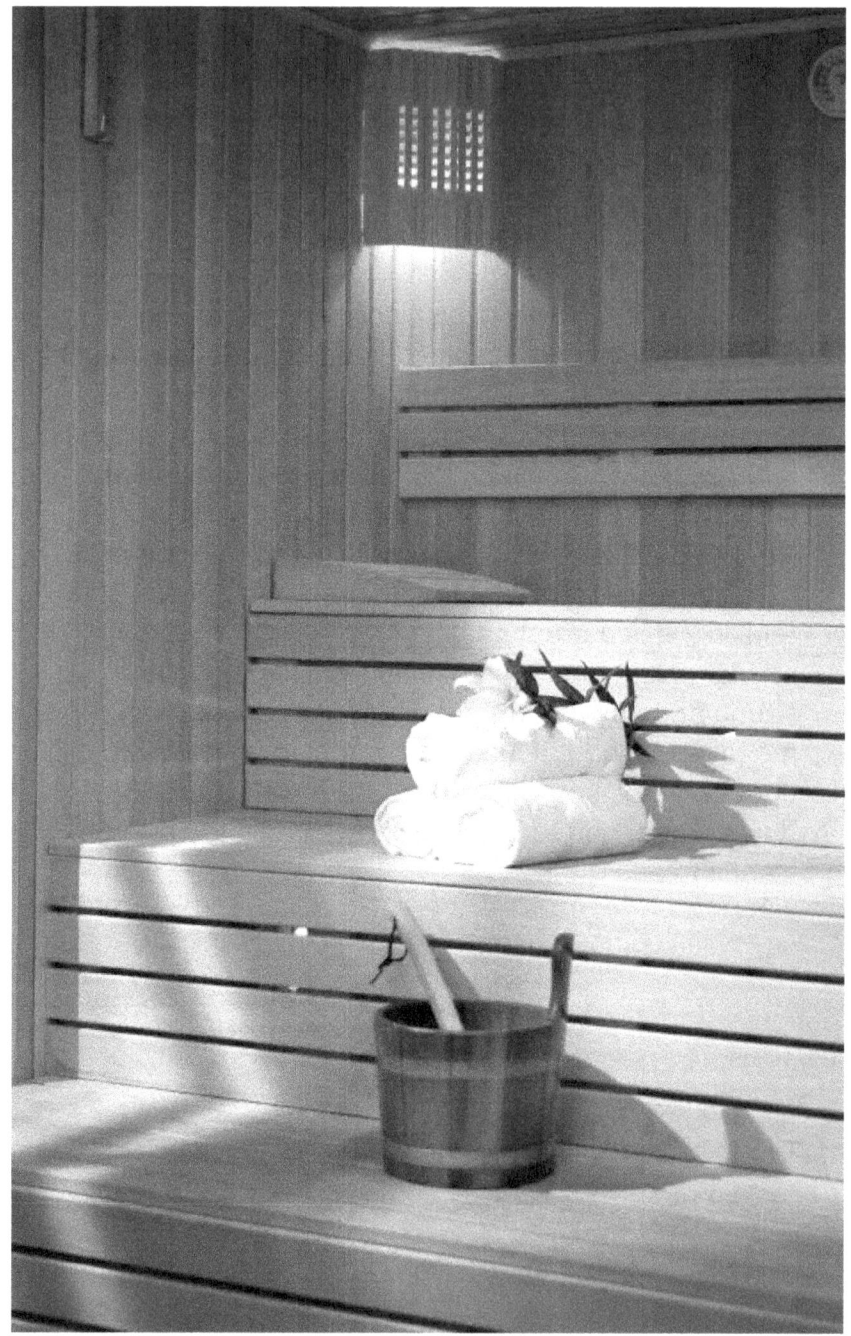

Step 10. Expect Failure

You are going to fail at this. Alot. You will use the picture of the person that you're using for motivation as a dart board. You will hear an old love song that will make you drown in your sorrow only to be comforted by a box of chocolates. There will be parties, and you will drink your allowed calories for the day easily in one hour. You will substitute your morning blueberry muffin for a cream filled donut with chocolate frosting. Rather than end your day with a serving of yogurt, you will head to the ice cream stand and devour a hot fudge sundae with extra whip cream. You will go out to dinner after 6:00 p.m. You are going to sit in your air conditioned house and laugh at the suggestion of me telling you to go sit in a 120 degree sauna for twenty minutes. You are going to give up, decide this whole plan is stupid, and go back to your old ways.

But deep down, you know this time is different. You truly want change to occur. You know my plan works. I am living proof. There are no excuses. Look at that picture that is motivating you, and know that this time, your dream is going to become a reality. You hold all the power. You are in control. You can do this. You will do this.

You are doing this. A setback? Nope. It's all part of the plan. The days that you fail make you realize how badly you want to succeed. Don't be discouraged, get encouraged. As you get used to this plan, your days of failure will be less. Your days of victory will be more.

Change is starting to happen in you. You will become the person you

know you were meant to be. This time, you're going to win. You're dream is going to come true.

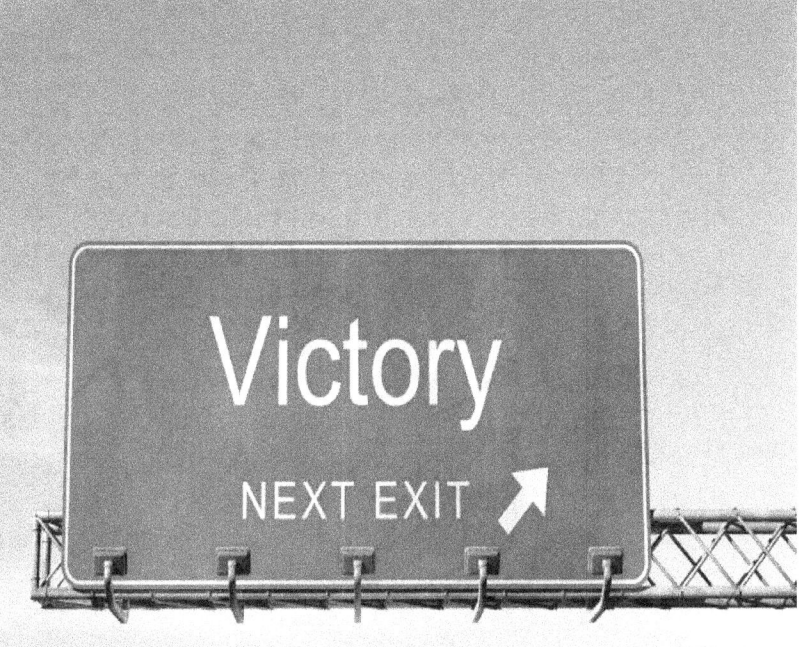

This may seem ridiculously short and simple to you. I could fill fifty more pages with "fluff" just to make this book longer so you feel like you really got your money's worth. But let's face it, all you care about is the ten things you need to do to lose weight. My goal is not to write a long, drawn out novel that I can charge $40.00 for and you will basically have to skip through to get to the part that is important. My goal is to teach you how to lose weight. These ten steps are all you need to know. These ten steps are the important parts. You never have to worry about being heavy again. I know it works. It worked for me and it continues to work for me today. It will work for you and continue to work for you for the rest of your life.

Everyday of your life you are faced with choices. Choices are opportunities. Opportunities make you benefit. You are going to benefit from your life choices. You are going to live the life you envision yourself living. You are going to become the person you envision yourself being. Starting today, you are going to make choices that benefit you. Starting today, you are in control. You are going to control where you go. You are going to the place of your dreams. You will become the person you dream of being.

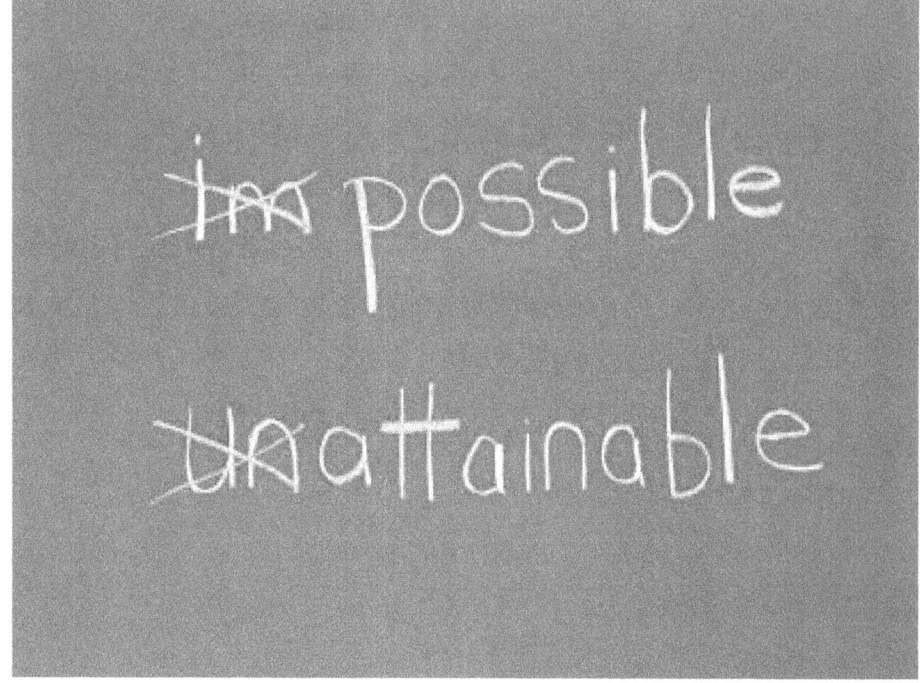

10 Step Plan

1. VISUALIZE THE END RESULT

2. LOSE WEIGHT INSTANTLY

3. THINK OF YOUR LIFE IN CALENDAR FORMAT

4. THINK LIKE A SOLDIER

5. DISCOVER YOUR NEW FAVORITE NUMBER

6. KEEP TRACK OF WHAT YOU CONSUME

7. EAT BLUEBERRIES AND YOGURT

8. DON'T EAT AFTER 6:00 P.M.

9. SIT IN A SAUNA FOR AT LEAST 20 MINUTES EVERYDAY

10. EXPECT FAILURE

I have provided a template on the following page as an example of one way to track your calories each day. I have found it is helpful to break up each day into four three hour intervals. Rather than think of a day as 12 hours and having an option of eating every hour, think of it as 4 time periods, and each time period you can consume a portion of your allowed calories.

6 am-9 am

food	calories
Total	

9 am-12 pm

food	calories
6 am-9 am Total	
Total	

12 pm-3 pm

food	calories
6 am-12 pm Total	
Total	

3 pm-6 pm

food	calories
Total	
6 am-3 pm Total	
DAY TOTAL	

33

In case you're wondering, my "favorite number" is 1254. I am 5'5" and weigh 114 pounds. I have been 114 for six years now since I discovered this ten step process. The heaviest I ever weighed was 190 pounds. The lightest I've ever been is 103 pounds. It is not advised to go under 1200 calories for women and 1800 calories for men.

People always ask me what I eat. I eat anything I am hungry for, but in moderation. I never feel "starved" or "deprived". Here is a sample of my diet on an average day.

6-9 am:	Nutz over Chocolate Luna® Bar	180 calories
9am – 12 noon:	Blueberry Muffin	350 calories
12-3pm:	Peanut Butter & Jelly Sandwich	
	(wheat bread)	300 calories
	Tostitos® Nachos	150 calories
3pm-6pm	(2) Weight Watchers® English Toffee	
	Crunch Ice Cream Bars	200 calories
6pm	Trix® yogurt	free
	TOTAL:	1180 calories
(coffee w/cream & sugar throughout day)		50 calories
		1230 calories

Initially, exercise is not required with my ten step plan. Focus first on getting your eating under control. Once you feel confident that you have control of your eating, you can introduce exercise into your daily routine if you want to. To lose weight, getting your eating under control is way more important than exercising. You do not have to exercise to lose weight. You do have to modify your diet to lose weight. If you exercise, then you can increase your calories per day to match the amount that you burned with activity.   Since your age and weight affect the amount of calories you burn, use a treadmill or elliptical. This way you can enter in your specific data and get a more accurate number for the amount of calories burned. If you have the option of exercising at night, I would advise you to do so. Since you can't eat after 6:00p.m., go to the gym, workout, then go in the sauna. By the time you get home, it will be time for bed and you won't have to worry about being tempted to snack. Don't think of exercise as a dreaded chore. Exercise is like a magic carpet. Once you hop on it, it is going to take you wherever you want to go. Where you want to go is as far away from where you are now as possible. You decide where you want to go. You decide how you want to look. You determine how much weight you're going to lose. You are in control. You are going to make change happen.

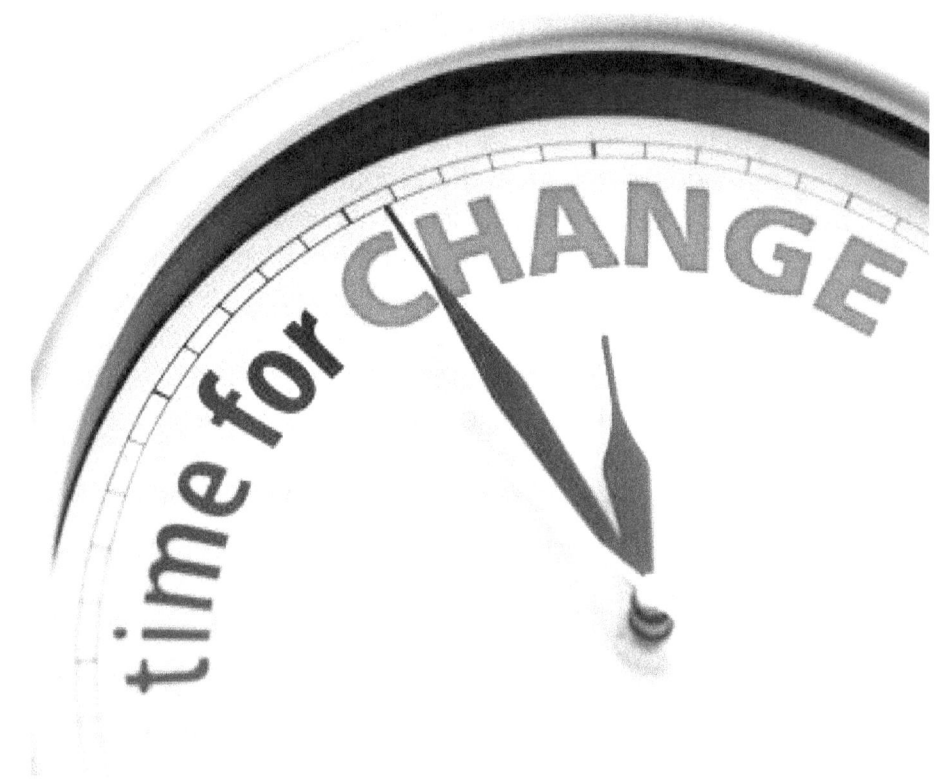

Let me be the first to congratulate you on your achievement.

Enjoy the new you. Keep being the best you can be and don't ever stop moving forward. Once you have reached your goal, you will feel like doing the things you always wanted to do. You will be bursting with joy and want to share it with the world. Do exactly that.

Whatever it is that you have to offer to the world, whatever you can do to help improve someone's life, do it. Keep the cycle of good going strong and always pay forward whatever it is you can to help someone else. Please email me when you start making progress and start seeing results. I would love to hear your success story!

LoriKnoble@2bskinny.com

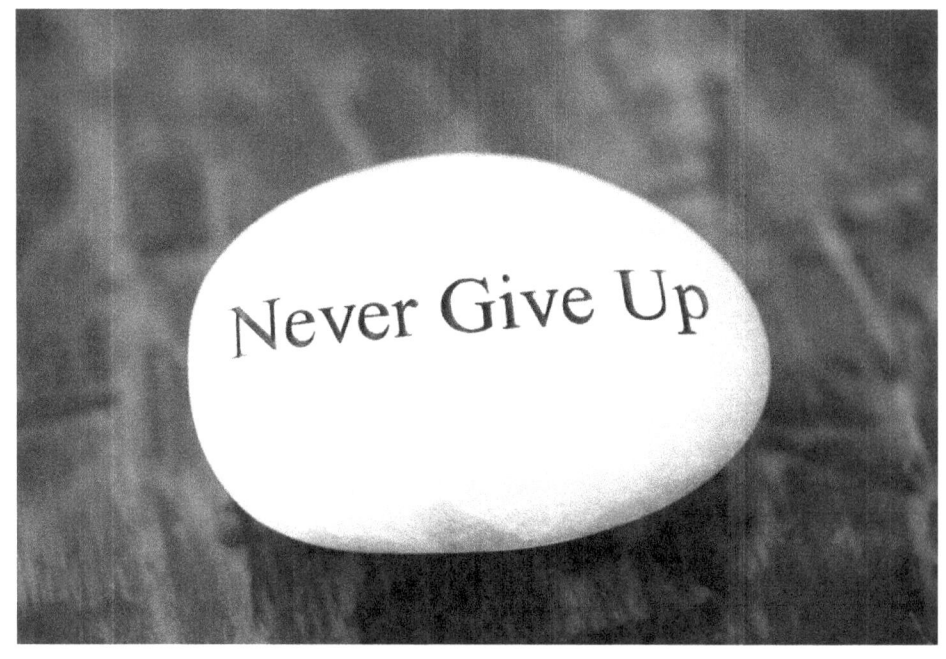

<u>My favorite quotes by Joel Osteen:</u>

"Be the one to stand out in the crowd."

"Your best days are still out in front of you"

"People of excellence go the extra mile to do what's right."

"You will never change what you tolerate."

"Do all you can to make your dreams come true."

"Don't just accept whatever comes your way in life. You were born to win; you were born for greatness; you were created to be a champion in life."

"Be a victor, not a victim."

39

<u>No Commercial Use</u>

I am the sole copyright owner of the information contained in this guide. You can share it with a friend that you know personally but you cannot distribute this guide or a part of this guide in any form to people you don't know personally – whether for free or for sale. You may not represent this guide as your own.

40

www.ingramcontent.com/pod-product-compliance
Lightning Source LLC
Chambersburg PA
CBHW070135290526
45789CB00011B/2209